Introduction

Drinking herbal tea has many benefits for your health! There are infinite number of ways to make delicious tea.

It is frugal to make teas from bulk herbs found in most herbal specialty stores. You can make teas from bulk herbs found in herbal specialty stores. Herbal teas are even more delicious when you infuse them with fruits or milk, add some honey or juice. And remember, they are natural!

This book contains a variety of recipes how you can make delicious tea. The book provides 80 recipes for you! Try some hot tea blends today and treat yourself, your friends and beloved ones!

1 Aromatic Tea

Ingredients

- 2 cups water
- 1 teaspoon powdered ginger
- 1 teaspoon powdered mint
- 1 teaspoon powdered turmeric
- 1 orange, juiced
- honey (optional)

Instructions

1. Boil 2 cups of water.
2. Remove pan from burner and add 1 teaspoon each of powdered spices. Stir, cover and let sit for 15-20 minutes.
3. Juice one orange and add to each cup.
4. The tea is ready.

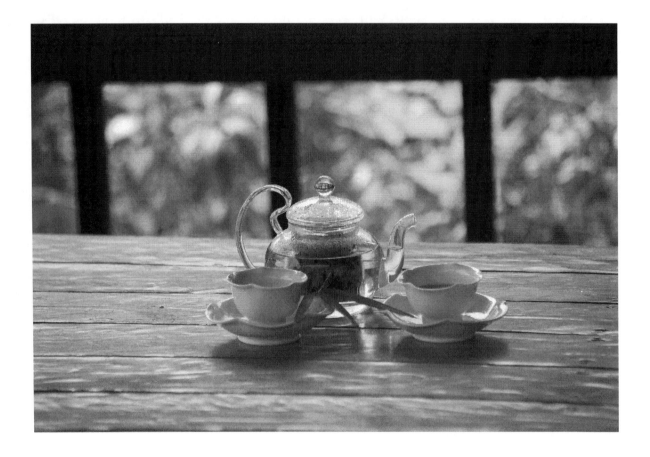

2 Cool Tea

Ingredients

- 3 cups water
- ½ teaspoon elderberries
- ½ teaspoon chamomile
- ½ teaspoon mint
- ½ teaspoon astragalus
- ½ teaspoon echinacea
- honey (optional)

Instructions

1. Boil 3 cups of water.
2. Remove pan from burner and add ½ teaspoon each of herb. Stir, cover and let sit for 20 minutes.
3. Add some honey.
4. The tea is ready.

3 Fragrant Tea

Ingredients

- 2 cups water
- 1 tablespoon of dried elderberry
- 1 cinnamon stick
- 3 whole cloves
- honey (optional)

Instructions

1. Boil 2 cups of water.
2. Remove pan from burner and add each of herb. Stir, cover and let sit for 20 minutes.
3. Add some honey.
4. The tea is ready.

4 Cold Tea

Ingredients

- 3 cups water
- 1 teaspoon powdered mint
- 1 teaspoon powdered turmeric
- 1 teaspoon lemon peel
- honey (optional)

Instructions

1. Boil 3 cups of water.
2. Remove pan from burner and add each of herb. Stir, cover and let sit for 10 minutes.
3. Add some honey.
4. The tea is ready.

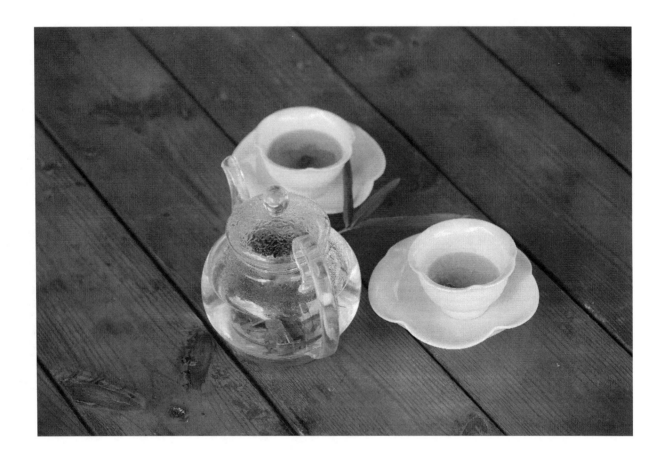

5 Winter Tea

Ingredients

- 3 cups water
- 1 cinnamon stick
- ½ teaspoon ground nutmeg
- ½ teaspoon ginger
- 3 whole cloves
- 1 teaspoon lemon peel
- honey (optional)

Instructions

1. Boil 3 cups of water.
2. Remove pan from burner and add each of herb. Stir, cover and let sit for 15 minutes.
3. Add some honey.
4. The tea is ready.

6 Fresh Tea

Ingredients

- 5 cups water
- 5 teaspoons black tea
- 8 black peppercorns
- 8 cloves
- 3 cinnamon sticks
- 1 star anise
- ½ inch fresh ginger
- ½ vanilla bean
- 1 teaspoon lemon peel
- honey (optional)

Instructions

1. Take a medium sized pot, boiled 5 cups of water.
2. Add to water peppercorns, cloves, cinnamon sticks, anise, black tea, ginger, vanilla and lemon peel. Simmer for 20 minutes.
3. Add some honey, if desired.
4. The concentrate will stay fresh in the fridge for up to 5 days. When ready to drink mix one part of tea with one part water or raw milk.

7 Pleasant Tea

Ingredients

- ½ teaspoon black peppercorn
- ½ teaspoon coriander seed
- 4 cloves
- 5 cm stick of cinnamon
- 1 teaspoon crystallised ginger, chopped
- 2 teaspoons black tea
- 1 orange
- honey (optional)

Instructions

1. Boil 3 cups of water.
2. Crush spices using a mortar and pestle. Remove pan from burner and add each of herb. Place spices with ginger   and black tea in a bowl and mix well. Stir, cover and let sit for 15 minutes. Then strain.
3. Add boiled water, some honey and orange to taste.

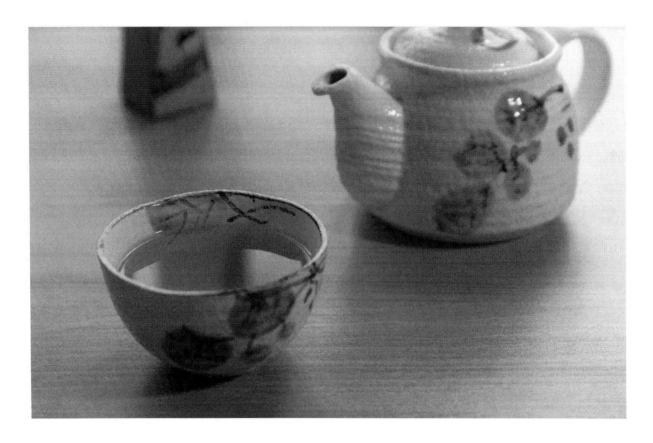

8 Autumn Tea

Ingredients

- ½ teaspoon nettle leaf
- ½ teaspoon spearmint leaf
- ½ teaspoon lemon balm
- lemon to taste
- ½ teaspoon red clover blossom
- ½ teaspoon rose hips
- ginger root to taste
- honey (optional)

Instructions

1. Boil 2 cups of water.
2. Crush spices using a mortar and pestle. Remove pan from burner and add each of herb. Place spices with ginger in a bowl and mix well. Stir, cover and let sit for 10 minutes. Then strain.
3. Add boiled water and some honey.

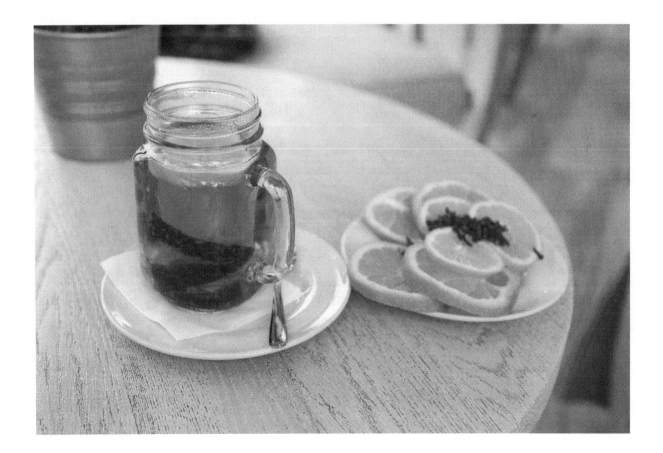

9 Healthy Tea

Ingredients

- 1 tablespoon rose hips
- 1 tablespoon cinnamon chips
- 1 teaspoon hibiscus flowers
- 1 teaspoon fennel seeds
- ½ teaspoon lemon peel
- 3 cups filtered water
- honey (optional)

Instructions

1. Boil 3 cups of water.
2. Crush spices using a mortar and pestle. Remove pan from burner and add each of herb. Place spices in a bowl and mix well. Stir, cover and let sit for 10 minutes. Then strain.
3. Add boiled water, fruit juice and some honey.

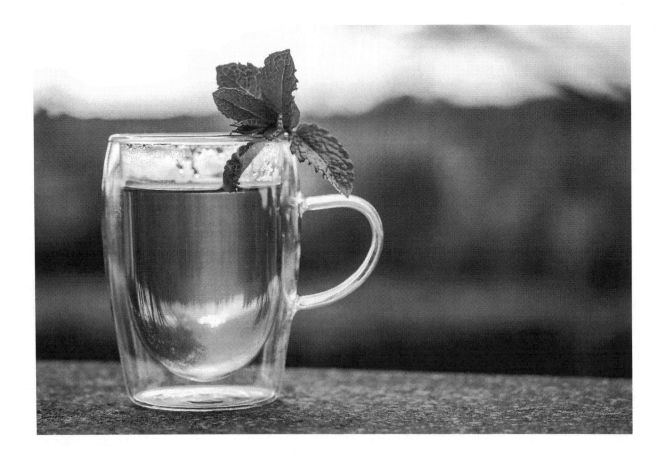

10 Summer Tea

Ingredients

- 1 sweet apple
- 2 teaspoons orange juice
- ½ teaspoon leaf black tea
- 5 whole cloves
- 1 cinnamon stick
- ½ teaspoon lemon peel
- honey (optional)

Instructions

1. Boil 3 cups of water.
2. Crush spices using a mortar and pestle. Slice the apple as thin as possible. Remove pan from burner and add each of herb. Place spices with apple in a bowl and mix well. Stir, cover and let sit for 10 minutes. Then strain.
3. Add boiled water, fruit juice and some honey.
4. The tea is ready.

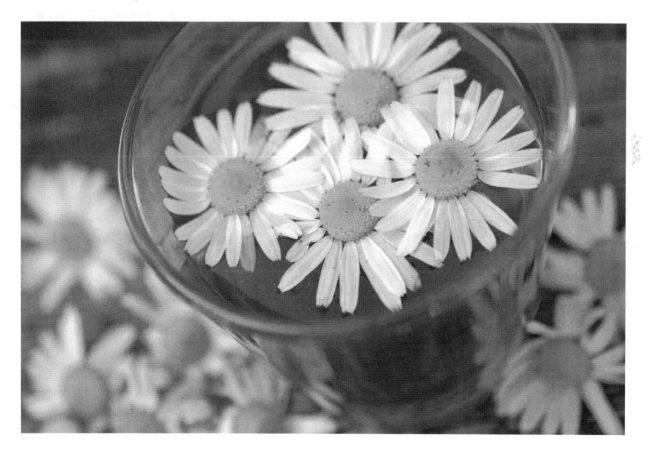

11 Eastern Tea

Ingredients

- 1 tablespoon spearmint leaves
- 4 g dried licorice root
- 1 teaspoon hibiscus flowers
- ½ teaspoon lemon peel
- honey (optional)

Instructions

1. Boil 3 cups of water.
2. Crush spices using a mortar and pestle. Remove pan from burner and add each of herb. Place spices and herbs in a bowl and mix well. Stir, cover and let sit for 10 minutes. Then strain.
3. Add boiled water, fruit juice and some honey.
4. The tea is ready.

12 Soft Tea

Ingredients

- 1 tablespoon dried peppermint
- ½ teaspoon lemon peel
- honey (optional)

Instructions

1. Boil 2 cups of water.
2. Crush spices using a mortar and pestle. Remove pan from burner and add each of herb. Place spices and herbs in a bowl and mix well. Stir, cover and let sit for 5 minutes. Then strain.
3. Add boiled water, fruit juice and some honey.
4. The tea is ready.

13 Homemade Tea

Ingredients

- 4 cups water
- ½ lemon juice
- ½ orange juice
- 2 tablespoons honey
- 5 whole cloves
- 1 teaspoon hibiscus flowers

Instructions

1. In a large saucepan, combine the 4 cups of hot water, lemon juice, orange juice, honey, hibiscus flowers and cloves. Bring to a boil.
2. Remove from heat. Allow steeping 3 minutes.
3. Pour through a strainer into 4 tea cups.
4. The tea is ready.

14 Milk Tea

Ingredients

- 250 g milk
- 2 teaspoons black tea
- ½ teaspoon fresh ginger
- 5-6 pieces carnation
- 250 g water
- honey (optional)

Instructions

1. Pour milk and water into the pot, put it on the fire and wait for the boiling.
2. Peeled root of ginger and rub on a small grater.
3. When milk boils, add tea. Reduce the heat to a minimum, stay for about 1 minute.
4. Add ginger. Turn it off and cover. Allow steeping 3 minutes.
5. Filter tea through a fine sieve. Add honey.
6. The tea is ready.

15 Delicious Tea

Ingredients

- 1 teaspoon hibiscus flowers
- ½ teaspoon lemon peel
- ½ cup cinnamon chips
- honey (optional)

Instructions

1. Blend all ingredients in a bowl.
2. Place 2 tablespoons of herb mix in a medium saucepan.
3. Pour 1-2 cups of hot water over herbs.
4. Bring to a quick boil and lower heat.
5. Allow to simmer 10-15 minutes.
6. Strain, and sweeten.

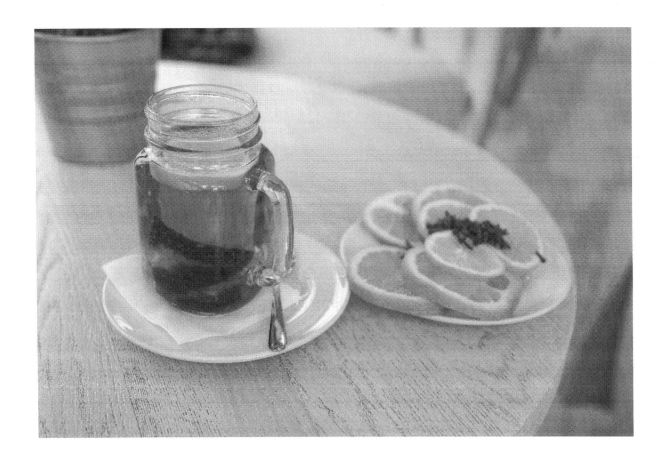

16 Tasty Tea

Ingredients

- 4 parts nettle leaf
- 3 parts spearmint leaves
- 2 parts red clover blossoms
- 1 part rose hips
- 1 part Ginger Root (dried, cut)
- honey (optional)

Instructions

1. Combine all the dry ingredients and store in a cool dry place.
2. To brew, boil 4 cups of water and pour that water over the tea blend.
3. Let it steep for 30 minutes, strain the herbs out.
4. Sweeten as desired.

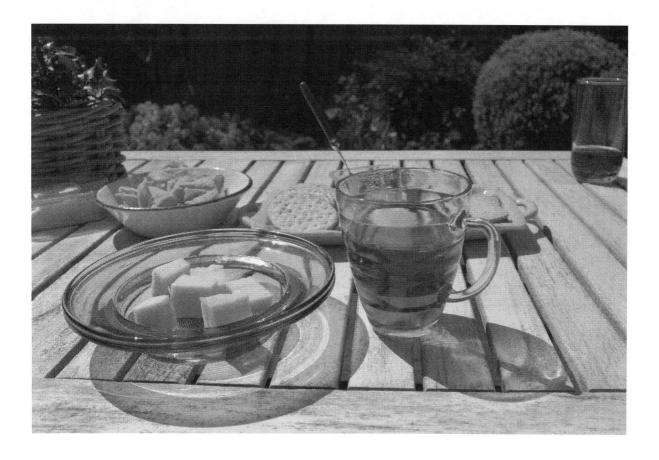

17 Warm Tea

Ingredients

- ¼ cup dried peppermint leaves
- ¼ cup dried spearmint leaves
- honey (optional)

Instructions

1. Combine all the dry ingredients.
2. Use one teaspoon of tea for a single serving.
3. Add 1 cup of boiled water.
4. Let it steep for 10 minutes, strain the herbs out.
5. Sweeten as desired.

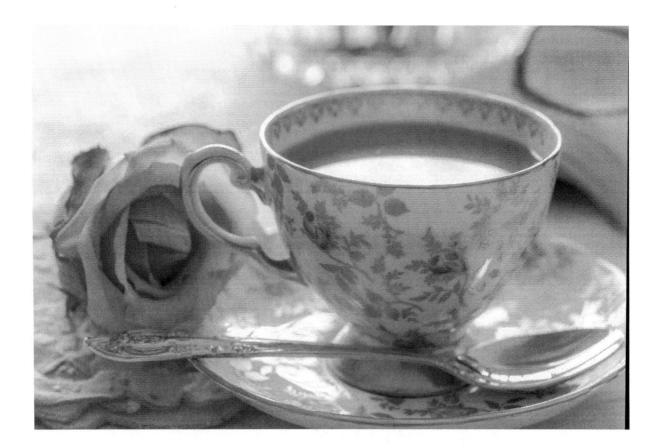

18 Astonished Tea

Ingredients

- 2 parts rose petals
- 1 part black tea
- honey (optional)

Instructions

1. Combine all the dry ingredients.
2. Usc onc tcaspoon of tca for a singlc scrving.
3. Pour 250 ml of boiling water over the tea.
4. Let it steep for 10 minutes, strain the herbs out.
5. Sweeten as desired.

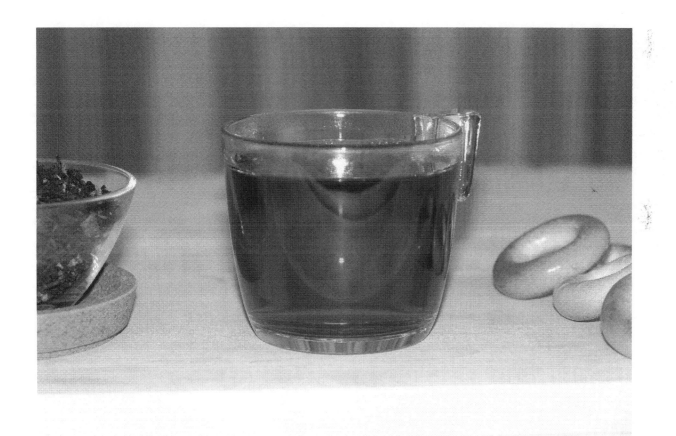

19 Tranquil Tea

Ingredients

- 4 parts chamomile
- 2 parts lemon grass
- 2 parts rose petals
- honey (optional)

Instructions

1. Add all the herbs to a glass jar and shake until they are completely mixed.
2. Use one teaspoon of tisane for a single serving. Add your desired amount to a tea strainer or teapot. Cover with boiling water a let steep for at least 5 minutes or up to 10.
3. Add some honey.

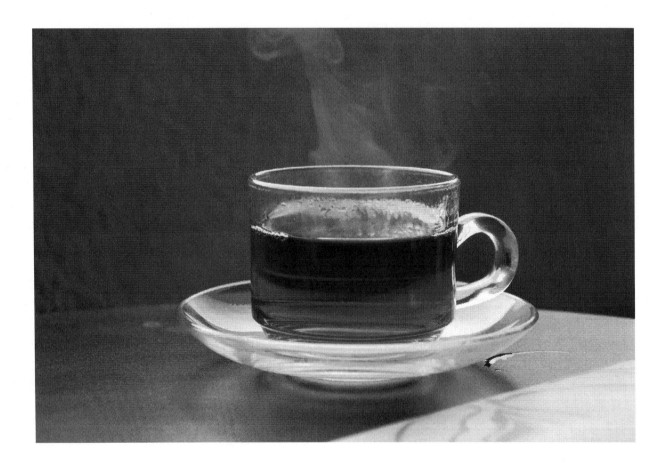

20 Cheery Tea

Ingredients

- 2 parts lemon grass
- 1 part lemon balm
- 1 part lemon peel
- 1 part chamomile
- 1 part cut stevia leaves
- honey (optional)

Instructions

1. Add all the herbs to a glass jar and shake until they are completely mixed.
2. Use one teaspoon of herbs for a single serving. Add your desired amount to a tea strainer or teapot.
3. Cover with boiling water a let steep for at least 5 minutes or up to 10.
4. Sweeten with honey if desired.

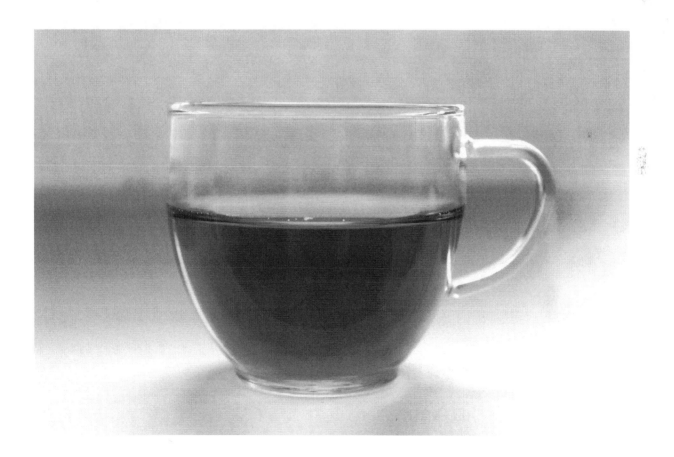

21 Delightful Tea

Ingredients

- 1 cup unsweetened coconut milk
- 1 cup water
- 1 black tea bag
- 1 tablespoon cocoa powder
- 1 part lemon peel
- honey (optional)

Instructions

1. Bring the coconut milk and water to a boil.
2. Steep the tea bags in the mixture for about 4 to 5 minutes.
3. Mix the cocoa powder and lemon peels together.
4. Remove the tea bags and stir in the cocoa mixture then pour it in cups.

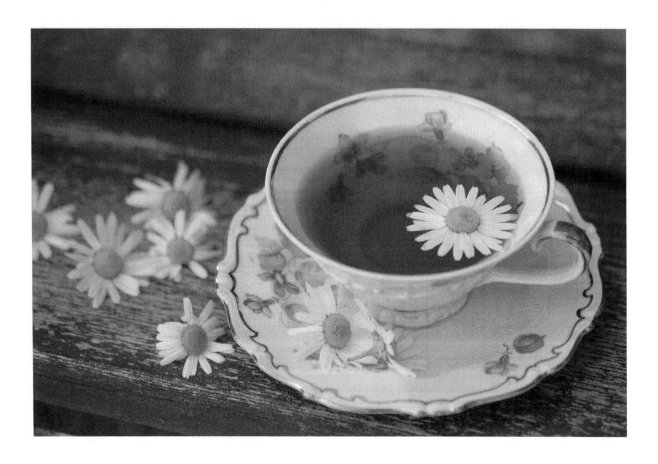

22 Excellent Tea

Ingredients

- 3 teaspoons cardamom
- 3 teaspoons cinnamon
- 1 teaspoon ground cloves
- 1 teaspoon nutmeg
- 2 teaspoons ground ginger
- honey (optional)

Instructions

1. Use one teaspoon of herbs for a single serving. Add your desired amount to a tea strainer or teapot.
2. Cover with boiling water a let steep for at least 5 minutes or up to 10.
3. Sweeten with honey if desired.

23 Good Tea

Ingredients

- ½ teaspoon nettle leaf
- ½ teaspoon spearmint leaf
- ½ teaspoon lemon balm
- honey (optional)

Instructions

1. 1 teaspoon dry herbs per cup of hot water.
2. Cover and let steep for at least 15 minutes.
3. Sweeten with honey.
4. Drink up to a quart warm or at room temperature throughout the day.

24 Happy Tea

Ingredients

- 1 teaspoon of cut dried red raspberry leaves
- ½ teaspoon of cut dried peppermint leaves
- honey (optional)

Instructions

1. Add dry herbs per cup of hot water.
2. Cover and let steep for at least 10 minutes.
3. Sweeten with honey.
4. Drink up to a quart warm or at room temperature throughout the day.

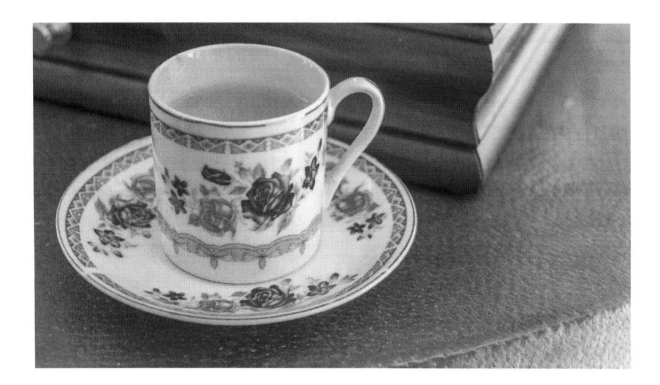

25 Joyful Tea

Ingredients

- 1 cup water
- ½ cup orange juice
- 1 teaspoon honey
- 1 teaspoon any black tea
- honey (optional)

Instructions

1. Add all ingredients per cup of hot water.
2. Cover and let steep for at least 10 minutes.
3. Drink up to a quart warm or at room temperature throughout the day.

26 Cheerful Tea

Ingredients

- 2 parts spearmint
- ¼ part peppermint
- 1 part chamomile
- ¼ part lemon balm
- ¼ part rose petals
- honey (optional)

Instructions

1. Mix all herbs in a large bowl.
2. To brew hot tea: Place 1 teaspoon tea per 1 cup boiling water.
3. Let steep 5-10 minutes and strain.
4. Sweeten with honey.

27 Optimistic Tea

Ingredients

- 1 tablespoon green tea
- 1 tablespoon chamomile
- 1 tablespoon hibiscus flowers
- 1 tablespoon orange peel
- honey (optional)

Instructions

1. Mix all herbs in a large bowl.
2. To brew hot tea: Place 1 teaspoon tea per 1 cup boiling water.
3. Let steep 5 minutes and strain.
4. Sweeten with honey.

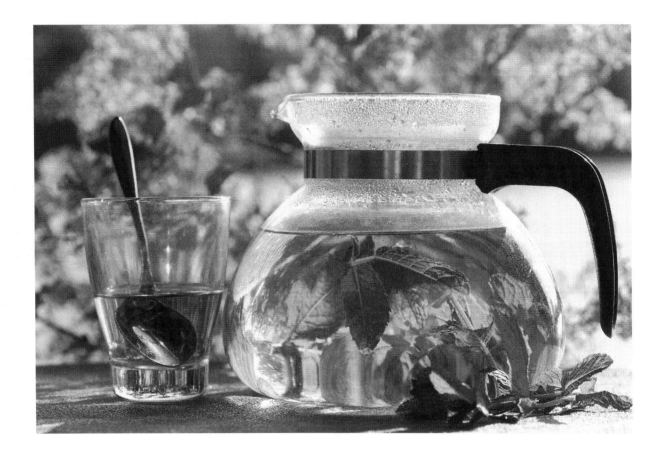

28 Vigorous Tea

Ingredients

- 1 tablespoon dried nettle leaf
- 2 tablespoons dried spearmint leaves
- 1 tablespoon dried green leaf stevia
- honey (optional)

Instructions

1. Mix all herbs in a large bowl.
2. To brew hot tea: Place 1 teaspoon tea per 1 cup boiling water.
3. Let steep 5 minutes and strain.
4. Sweeten with honey.
5. Drink 2 cups per day.

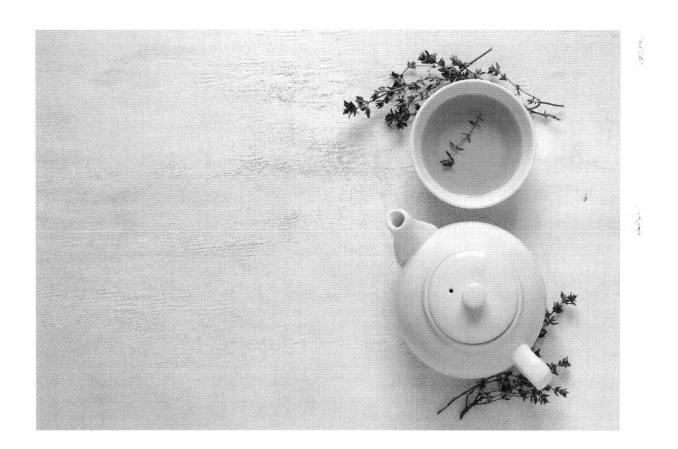

29 Purposeful Tea

Ingredients

- 1 cup fresh mint leaves
- ½ cup honey
- lemon to taste

Instructions

1. Put mint leaves and water into a sauce pan. Heat over medium heat for 30 min.
2. Take the sauce pan off the burner and allow it to cool.
3. Let steep 15 minutes and strain.
4. Add ½ cup of honey and stir and add some lemon to taste.

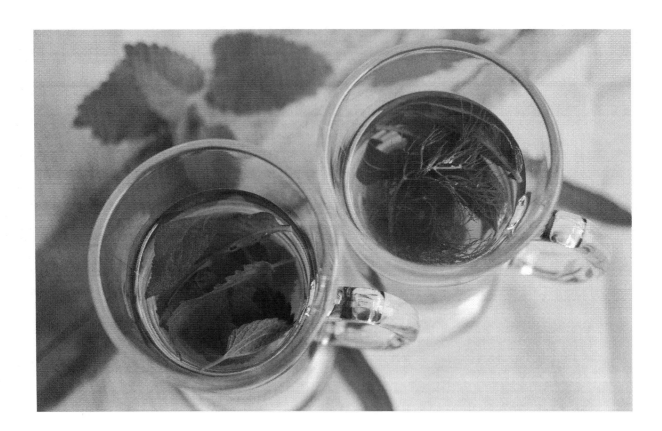

30 Respectful Tea

Ingredients

- 2 teaspoons cardamom
- 2 teaspoons cinnamon
- 1 teaspoon ground cloves
- ½ teaspoon nettle leaf
- ½ teaspoon spearmint leaf
- honey (optional)

Instructions

1. Mix all herbs in a large bowl.
2. To brew hot tea: Place 1 teaspoon tea per 1 cup boiling water.
3. Let steep 5 minutes and strain.
4. Sweeten with honey.

31 Correct Tea

Ingredients

- 1 tablespoon chamomile
- ½ tablespoon lavender
- ½ tablespoon catnip
- 1 tablespoon rose hips
- 1 tablespoon red clover
- honey (optional)

Instructions

1. Mix all herbs in a large bowl.
2. To brew hot tea: Place 1 teaspoon tea per 1 cup boiling water.
3. Let steep 5 minutes and strain.
4. Sweeten with honey.

32 Easy Tea

Ingredients

- 2 tablespoons chamomile
- 1 tablespoon St John's Wort
- 1 pinch lavender
- honey (optional)

Instructions

1. Mix all herbs in a large bowl.
2. To brew hot tea: Place 1 tablespoon tea per 1 cup boiling water.
3. Let steep 15 minutes and strain.
4. Sweeten with honey.

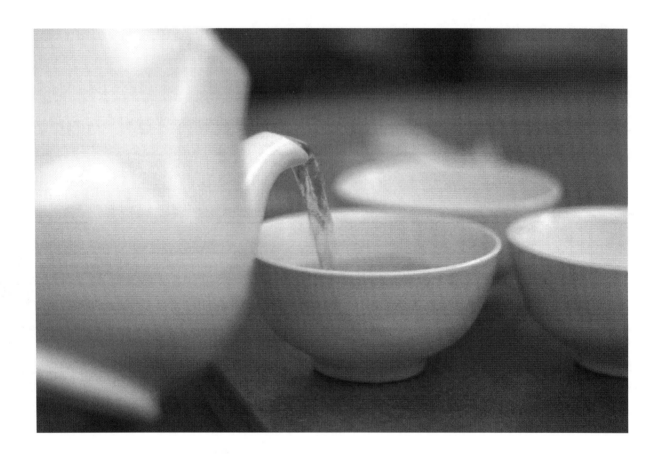

33 Natural Tea

Ingredients

- 2 to 5 cloves
- 4 to 8 cardamom pods
- 1 sticks cinnamon
- 1 nice size slices ginger root
- ½ teaspoon fennel seeds
- honey (optional)

Instructions

1. Smash all herbs in a mortar and pestle until they are busted open.
2. To brew hot tea: Place 1 teaspoon tea per 1 cup boiling water.
3. Let steep 20 minutes and strain.
4. Add honey to taste!

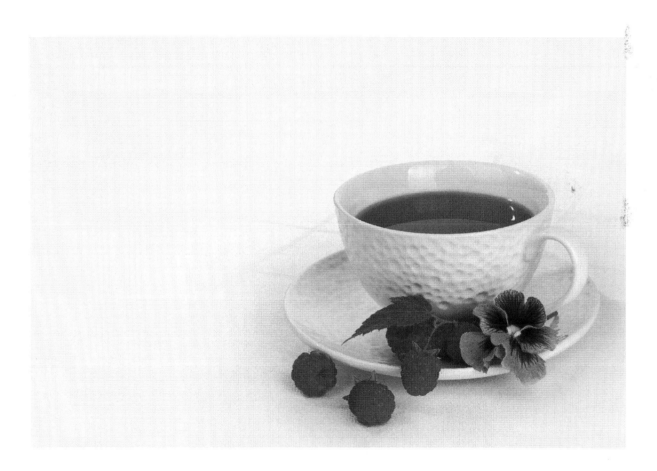

34 Reliable Tea

Ingredients

- 1 tablespoon peppermint
- 1 tablespoon lemon balm
- honey (optional)

Instructions

1. Mix all herbs in a large bowl.
2. To brew hot tea: Place 1 tablespoon tea per 1 cup boiling water.
3. Let steep 15 minutes or longer and strain.
4. Sweeten with honey.

35 Particular Tea

Ingredients

- 2 tablespoons lemon balm
- 1 tablespoon peppermint
- 1 tablespoon nettle
- 2 tablespoons rose hips
- honey (optional)

Instructions

1. Mix all herbs in a large bowl.
2. To brew hot tea: Place 1 tablespoon tea per 1 cup boiling water.
3. Let steep 15 minutes or longer and strain.
4. Sweeten with honey.

36 Positive Tea

Ingredients

- 5 whole, dried red hibiscus flowers
- ½ cup dried heavily scented rose petals
- ¼ cup fresh chopped rose hips
- 1 dried pear
- ½ cup dried black currants or elderberries
- 1 dried apricot
- 1 dried apple
- honey (optional)

Instructions

1. Chop finely all the fruit.
2. Mix all ingredients in a large bowl.
3. To brew hot tea: Place 1 tablespoon tea per 1 cup boiling water.
4. Let steep 15 minutes or longer and strain.
5. Sweeten with honey.

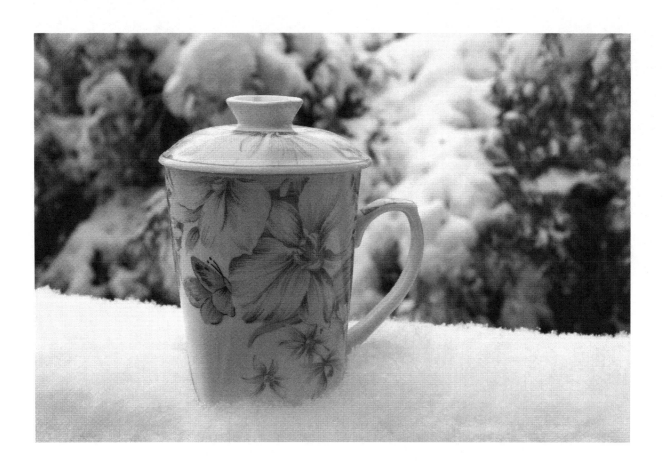

37 Lemon Tea

Ingredients

- ¼ cup lemon balm
- ¾ cup lemon grass
- honey to taste (optional)

Instructions

1. Mix all herbs in a large bowl.
2. To brew hot tea: Place 1 tablespoon tea per 1 cup boiling water.
3. Let steep 8 - 10 minutes and strain.
4. Sweeten with honey.

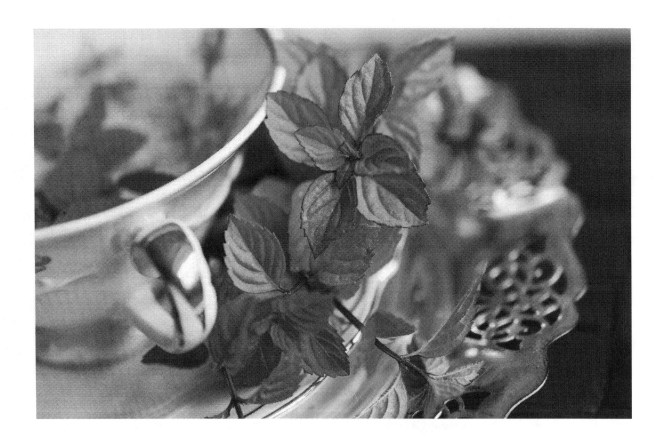

38 Real Tea

Ingredients

- 1 teaspoon dried peppermint leaves
- 1 teaspoon sugar or honey
- 1 cup of water

Instructions

1. To brew hot tea: Place 1 tablespoon tea per 1 cup boiling water.
2. Let steep 5 - 10 minutes and strain.
3. Sweeten with honey.

39 Lavender Tea

Ingredients

- 2 tablespoons fresh organic lavender
- ¼ cup dried mint
- 3 cups hot water

Instructions

1. Combine mint and lavender in a tea pot, add hot water.
2. Let it steep for at least 5 minutes and strain.
3. Add fresh lemon or honey to taste.

40 Special Tea

Ingredients

- ½ cup orange juice
- ½ cup lemon juice
- 4 cloves
- 2 stars anise
- ½ cinnamon stick for each cup
- ½ cup any black tea
- honey to taste (optional)

Instructions

1. Bring water to a boil (3 cups hot water).
2. Add all ingredients (except cinnamon stick) to tea strainer.
3. Let it steep for at least 15 minutes and strain.
4. Add cinnamon stick and sweeten with honey.

41 Rose Tea

Ingredients

- 2 cups organic rose petals
- 1 cup chamomile blossoms
- 2 cups lemon grass
- 1 pinch of lavender
- honey to taste (optional)

Instructions

1. Mix all ingredients in a large bowl.
2. To brew hot tea: Place 1 teaspoon tea per 1 cup boiling water.
3. Let steep 5 - 10 minutes and strain.
4. Sweeten with honey.

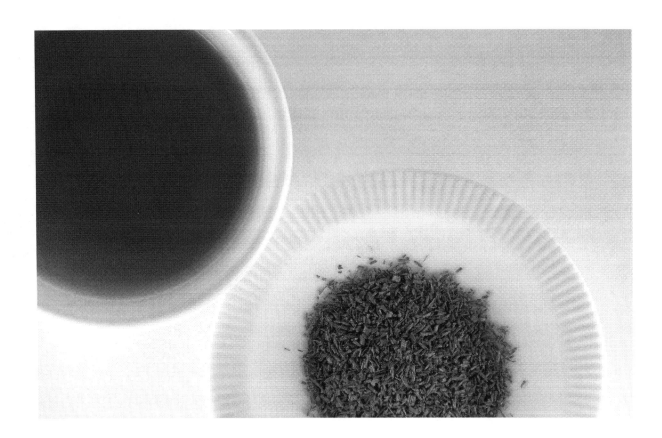

42 Useful Tea

Ingredients

- 1 tablespoon mint
- ¼ cup lemon balm
- 1 tablespoon red clover
- honey (optional)

Instructions

1. Mix all ingredients in a bowl.
2. To brew hot tea: Place 1 teaspoon tea per 1 cup boiling water.
3. Let steep 10 - 15 minutes and strain.
4. Sweeten with honey.

43 Clever Tea

Ingredients

- 2 cups lemon grass
- 1 pinch of lavender
- ¼ cup dried mint
- honey (optional)

Instructions

1. Mix all ingredients in a bowl.
2. To brew hot tea: Place 1 teaspoon tea per 1 cup boiling water.
3. Let steep 10 minutes and strain.
4. Sweeten with honey.

44 Gifted Tea

Ingredients

- 6 teaspoons green tea
- ½ teaspoon hibiscus blooms
- 2 oz. dried fruit or berries, crushed
- honey (optional)

Instructions

1. Mix all ingredients in a bowl.
2. To brew hot tea: Place 1 teaspoon tea per 1 cup boiling water.
3. Let steep 3 minutes and strain.
4. Sweeten with honey.

45 Great Tea

Ingredients

- 2 teaspoons cardamom
- 2 teaspoons cinnamon
- 1 teaspoon ground cloves
- 4 cloves
- 2 stars anise
- honey (optional)

Instructions

1. Mix all ingredients in a bowl.
2. To brew hot tea: Place 1 teaspoon tea per 1 cup boiling water.
3. Let steep 3 minutes and strain.
4. Sweeten with honey.

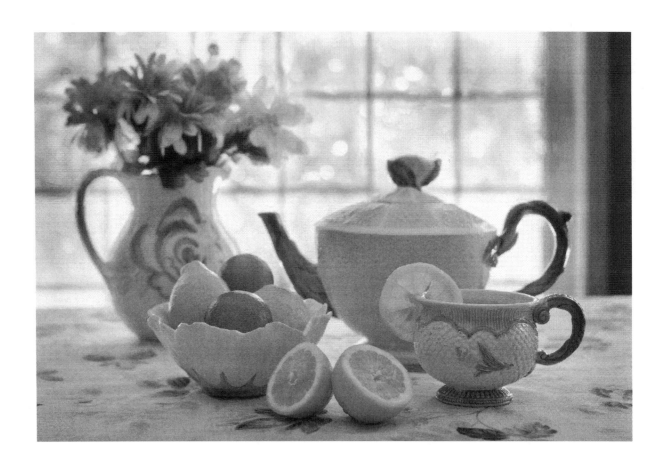

46 Ancient Tea

Ingredients

- 2 teaspoons cardamom
- 1 cup chamomile blossoms
- 4 cloves
- 2 stars anise
- honey (optional)

Instructions

1. Mix all ingredients in a bowl.
2. To brew hot tea: Place 1 teaspoon tea per 1 cup boiling water.
3. Let steep 20 minutes and strain.
4. Sweeten with honey.

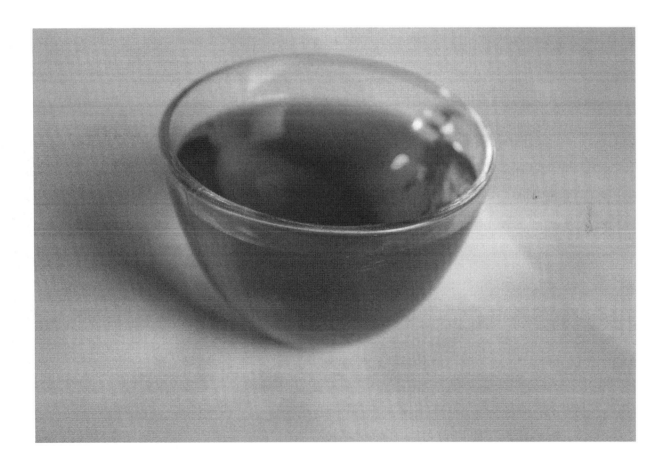

47 Constant Tea

Ingredients

- 1 teaspoon lavender
- 1 teaspoon of your favorite mint
- 1 teaspoon chamomile
- honey (optional)

Instructions

1. Mix all ingredients in a bowl.
2. Add 1 teaspoon of each of these herbs for every cup of tea.
3. Put herbs in a teapot and fill it with boiling water.
4. Let steep 10 minutes and strain.
5. Sweeten with honey.

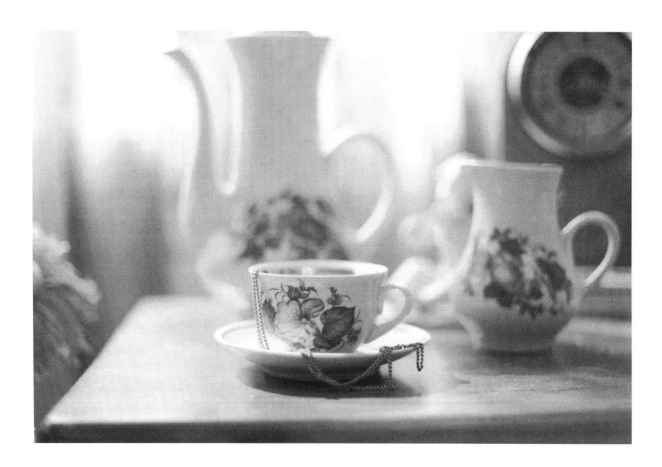

48 Early Tea

Ingredients

- 2 cups catnip
- 1 cup chamomile
- 1 cup lemon balm
- 2 stars anise
- honey (optional)

Instructions

1. Mix all ingredients in a bowl.
2. To brew hot tea: Place 1 teaspoon tea per 1 cup boiling water.
3. Let steep 5 minutes and strain.
4. Sweeten with honey.

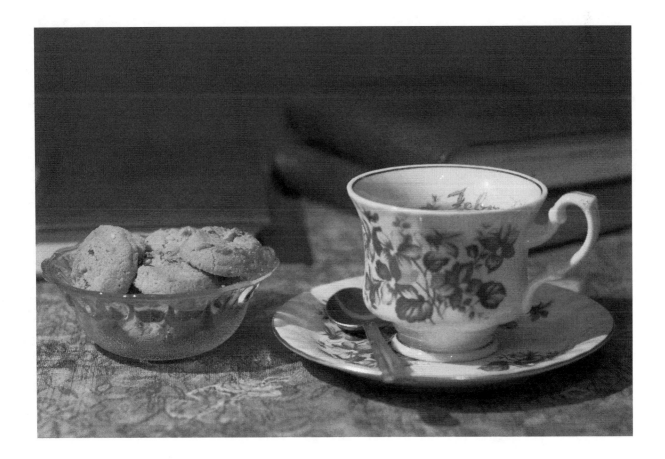

49 Fast Tea

Ingredients

- 4 tablespoons catnip
- 1 tablespoon red clover
- 4 tablespoons rose hips
- honey (optional)

Instructions

1. Mix all ingredients in a bowl.
2. To brew hot tea: Place 1 teaspoon tea per 1 cup boiling water.
3. Let steep 5 minutes and strain.
4. Sweeten with honey.

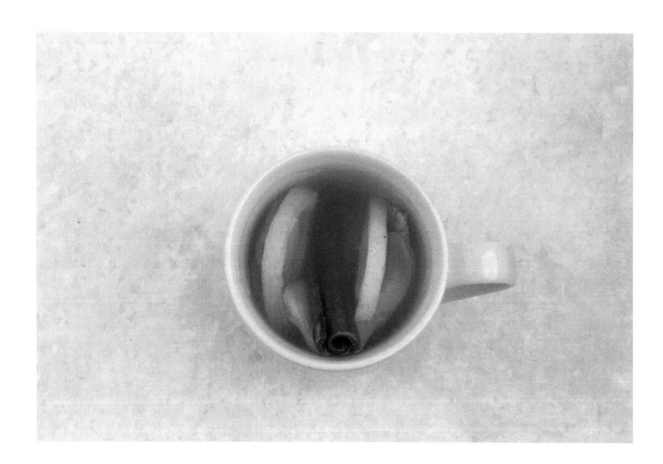

50 Present Tea

Ingredients

- 2 tablespoons rose hips
- ½ tablespoon chamomile
- 1 tablespoon nettle
- ½ tablespoon mints
- 1 tablespoon lemon balm
- honey (optional)

Instructions

1. Mix all ingredients in a bowl.
2. To brew hot tea: Place 1 teaspoon tea per 1 cup boiling water.
3. Let steep 5 minutes and strain.
4. Sweeten with honey.

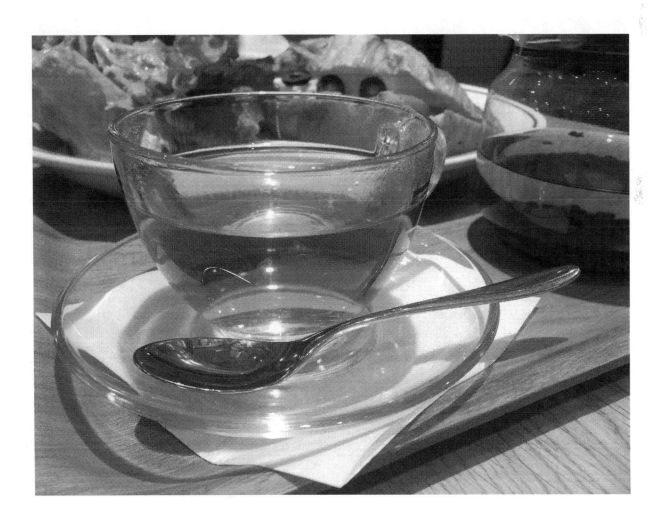

51 Spring Tea

Ingredients

- 1 cup black tea
- 1 teaspoon ground nutmeg
- 1 teaspoon ginger
- 1teaspoon cinnamon
- 1-2 chopped up vanilla beans
- honey (optional)

Instructions

1. Mix all ingredients in a bowl.
2. To brew hot tea: Place 1 teaspoon tea per 1 cup boiling water.
3. Let steep 7 minutes and strain.
4. Sweeten with honey.

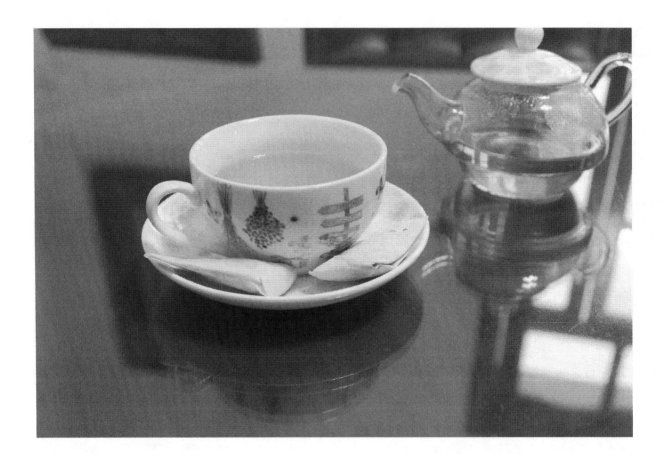

52 Granny Tea

Ingredients

- ½ teaspoon turmeric
- ¼ teaspoon ginger
- 1 teaspoon cinnamon
- honey (optional)

Instructions

1. Mix all ingredients in a bowl.
2. To brew hot tea: Place 1 teaspoon tea per 1 cup boiling water.
3. Let steep 15 minutes and strain.
4. Sweeten with honey.

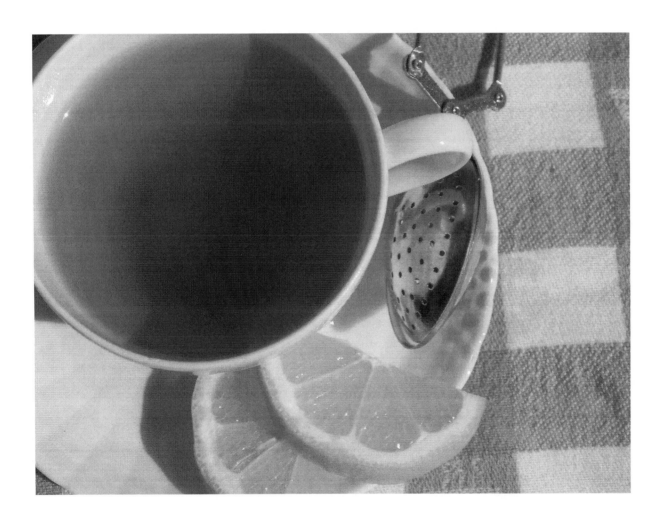

53 Expectant Tea

Ingredients

- 1 cup nettle
- 1 cup raspberry leaf
- 1 cup chamomile
- 1 cup lemon balm
- ½ cup lavender
- honey (optional)

Instructions

1. Mix all ingredients in a bowl.
2. To brew hot tea: Place 1 teaspoon tea per 1 cup boiling water.
3. Let steep 5 minutes and strain.
4. Sweeten with honey.

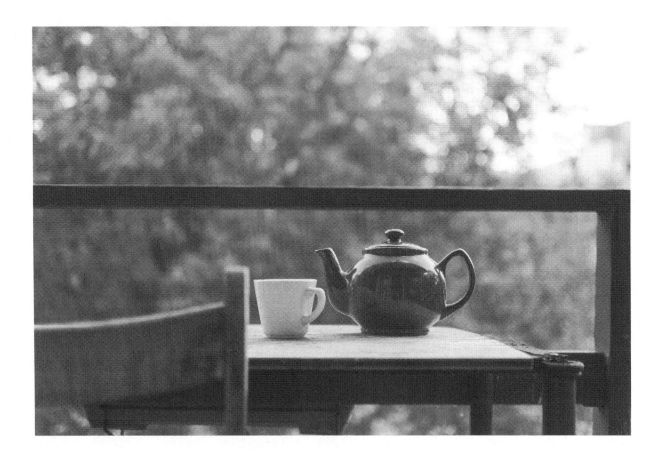

54 Nettle Tea

Ingredients

- 1 teaspoon nettle
- 1 teaspoon chamomile
- honey (optional)

Instructions

1. Mix all ingredients in a bowl.
2. To brew hot tea: Place 1 teaspoon tea per 1 cup boiling water.
3. Let steep 10 minutes and strain.
4. Sweeten with honey.

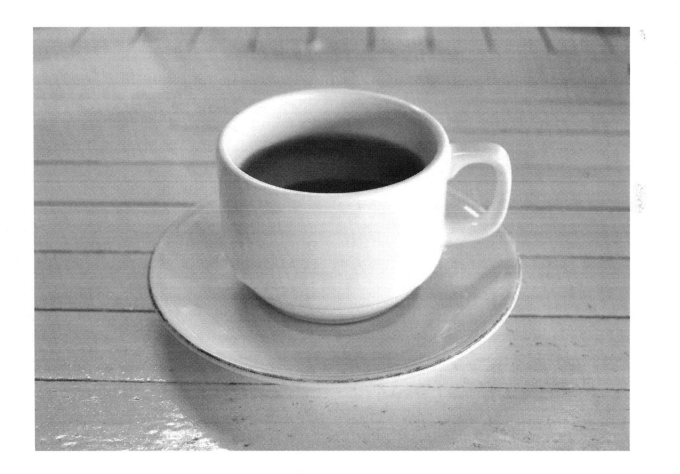

55 Yellow Tea

Ingredients

- 1 teaspoon organic lemon peel
- 1 teaspoon lemon balm
- 1 teaspoon chamomile
- 1 teaspoon skull cap
- ½ teaspoon lavender
- honey (optional)

Instructions

1. Mix all ingredients in a bowl.
2. To brew hot tea: Place 1 teaspoon tea per 1 cup boiling water.
3. Let steep 5 minutes and strain.
4. Sweeten with honey.

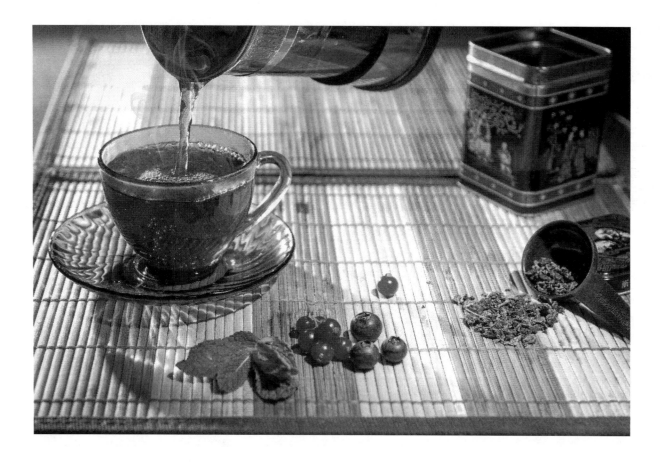

56 Nutritious Tea

Ingredients

- 1 cup of chopped oat straw
- 1 cup red raspberry leaves, chopped
- ½ cup dried peppermint leaves
- ½ tablespoon lavender
- honey (optional)

Instructions

1. Mix all ingredients in a bowl.
2. To brew hot tea: Place 1 teaspoon tea per 1 cup boiling water.
3. Let steep 8 - 10 minutes and strain.
4. Sweeten with honey.

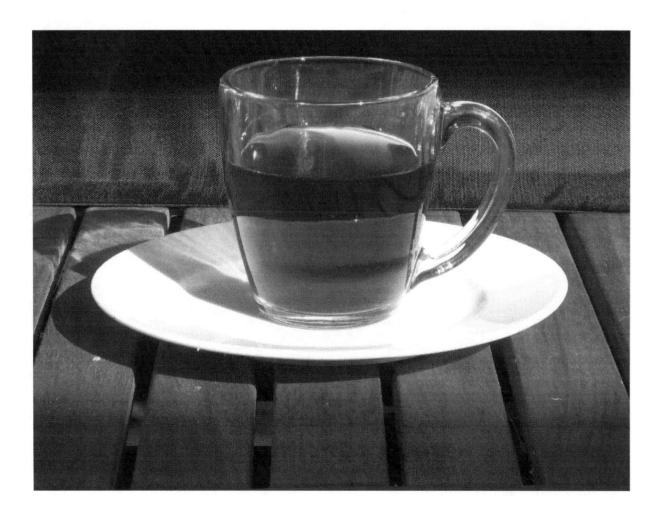

57 Ginger Tea

Ingredients

- 1 teaspoon ginger root, grated
- 1 ½ teaspoon honey
- 2 cloves
- 1-inch piece cinnamon bark
- 2-inch strip orange peel
- 1 star anise

Instructions

1. Mix all ingredients in a bowl.
2. To brew hot tea: Place 1 teaspoon tea per 1 cup boiling water.
3. Let steep 15 minutes and strain.
4. Sweeten with honey.

58 Pepper Tea

Ingredients

- ½ lemon juice
- ½ teaspoon turmeric powder
- ¼ teaspoon pepper
- 1 ½ teaspoon honey

Instructions

1. Place the pepper and turmeric in the cup, pour over boiling water.
2. Stir in the lemon juice and honey.

59 ABC Tea

Ingredients

- 3-inch piece dried ashwagandha root
- 2-inch strip orange peel
- 1 star anise
- honey (optional)

Instructions

1. Mix all ingredients in a bowl.
2. To brew hot tea: Place 1 teaspoon tea per 1 cup boiling water.
3. Let steep 20 minutes and strain.
4. Sweeten with honey.

60 Basil Tea

Ingredients

- ¼ cup basil
- 2 teaspoons lemon juice
- 1 star anise
- ½ teaspoon lavender
- honey (optional)

Instructions

1. Mix all ingredients in a bowl.
2. To brew hot tea: Place 1 teaspoon tea per 1 cup boiling water.
3. Let steep 15 minutes and strain.
4. Sweeten with honey.

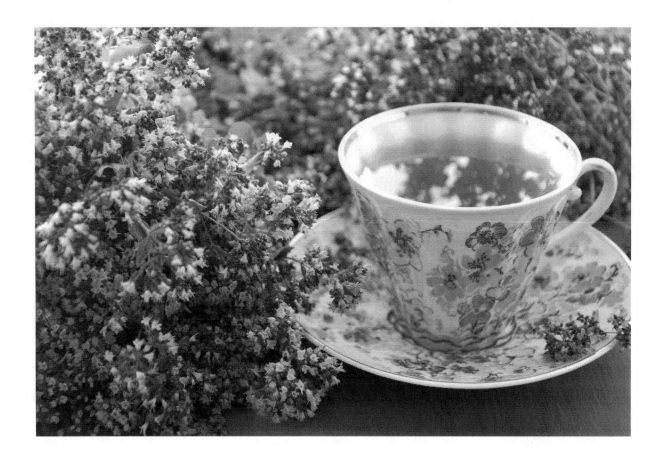

61 Mint Tea

Ingredients

- 15 mint leaves
- 1 sprig rosemary
- ½ teaspoon lavender
- honey (optional)

Instructions

1. Mix all ingredients in a bowl.
2. To brew hot tea: Place 1 teaspoon tea per 1 cup boiling water.
3. Let steep 5 minutes and strain.
4. Sweeten with honey.

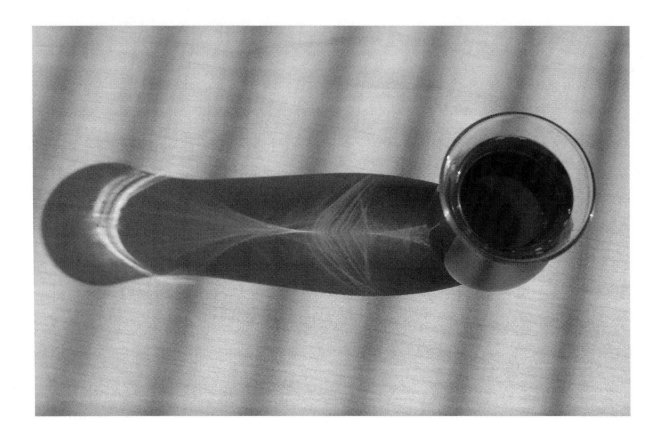

62 Southern Tea

Ingredients

- 1 cup spearmint
- 1 tablespoon black tea
- 1 teaspoon chamomile
- honey (optional)

Instructions

1. Mix all ingredients in a bowl.
2. To brew hot tea: Place 1 teaspoon tea per 1 cup boiling water.
3. Let steep 7 minutes and strain.
4. Sweeten with honey.

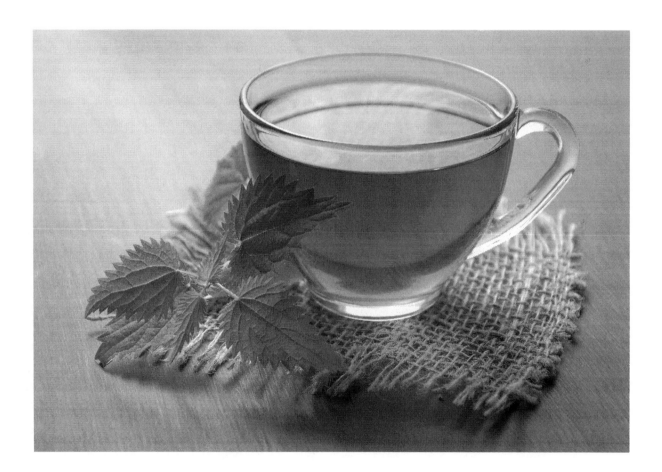

63 Northern Tea

Ingredients

- ½ part lemon balm
- ½ part lemon thyme
- ⅛ part lemon zest
- ¼ teaspoon lavender
- honey (optional)

Instructions

1. Mix all ingredients in a bowl.
2. To brew hot tea: Place 1 teaspoon tea per 1 cup boiling water.
3. Let steep 7 minutes and strain.
4. Sweeten with honey.

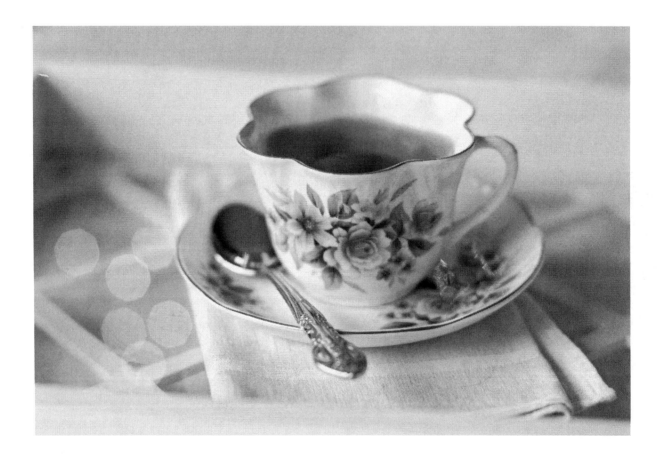

64 Eastern Tea

Ingredients

- 1 part chamomile
- 1 part red raspberry leaf
- ½ tablespoon catnip
- 1 tablespoon rose hips
- ¼ teaspoon lavender
- honey (optional)

Instructions

1. Mix all ingredients in a bowl.
2. To brew hot tea: Place 1 teaspoon tea per 1 cup boiling water.
3. Let steep 12 minutes and strain.
4. Sweeten with honey.

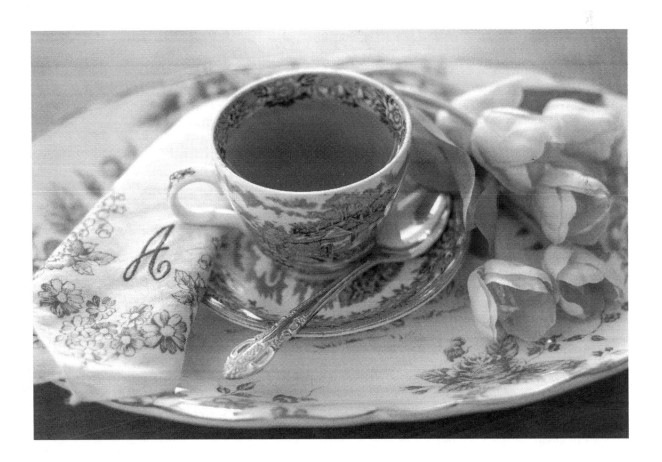

65 Western Tea

Ingredients

- 1 tablespoon anise hyssop
- 3 tablespoons spearmint
- 4 cloves
- honey (optional)

Instructions

1. Mix all ingredients in a bowl.
2. To brew hot tea: Place 1 teaspoon tea per 1 cup boiling water.
3. Let steep 10 minutes and strain.
4. Sweeten with honey.

66 White Tea

Ingredients

- 2 teaspoons peppermint leaf
- ½ teaspoon fennel seeds
- Pinch of dried ginger
- ¼ teaspoon lavender
- honey (optional)

Instructions

1. Mix all ingredients in a bowl.
2. To brew hot tea: Place 1 teaspoon tea per 1 cup boiling water.
3. Let steep 10 minutes and strain.
4. Sweeten with honey.

67 Berry Tea

Ingredients

- 1 cinnamon stick
- 2 cardamom pods
- honey (optional)

Instructions

1. Place all ingredients per 2 cups boiling water.
2. Let steep 30 minutes and strain.
3. Sweeten with honey.

68 Life Tea

Ingredients

- ½ cup rose petals
- ½ cup rosemary
- 1 tablespoon jasmine blossoms
- ½ cup hibiscus flowers
- honey (optional)

Instructions

1. Mix all ingredients in a bowl.
2. To brew hot tea: Place 1 teaspoon tea per 1 cup boiling water.
3. Let steep 10 minutes and strain.
4. Sweeten with honey.

69 Sage Tea

Ingredients

- ¼ cup dried basil leaves
- ½ teaspoon green tea
- ½ tablespoon chamomile
- honey (optional)

Instructions

1. Mix all ingredients in a bowl.
2. To brew hot tea: Place 1 teaspoon tea per 1 cup boiling water.
3. Let steep 10 minutes and strain.
4. Sweeten with honey.

70 Rosemary Tea

Ingredients

- 2 teaspoons dried rosemary
- ¼ cup dried mint
- honey (optional)

Instructions

1. Mix all ingredients in a bowl.
2. To brew hot tea: Place 2 teaspoons tea per 1 cup boiling water.
3. Let steep 10 minutes and strain.
4. Sweeten with honey.

71 Humorous Tea

Ingredients

- ½ cup cinnamon
- ½ teaspoon nutmeg
- ½ teaspoon cinnamon
- honey (optional)

Instructions

1. Mix all ingredients in a bowl.
2. To brew hot tea: Place 1 teaspoon tea per 1 cup boiling water.
3. Let steep 6 minutes and strain.
4. Sweeten with honey.

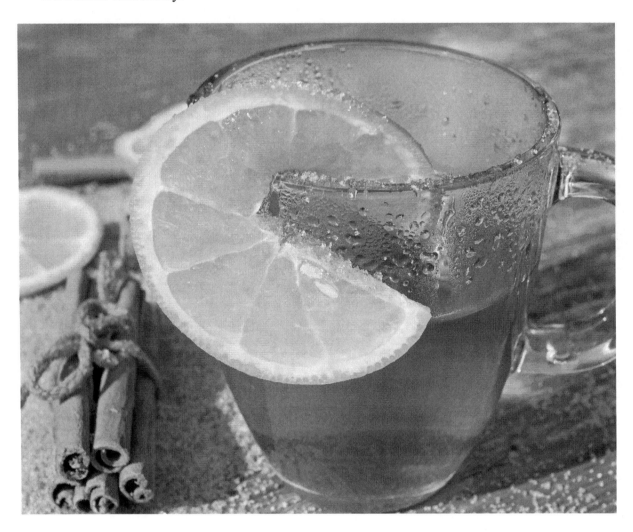

72 Memory Tea

Ingredients

- 1 cup dried rose petals
- 1 tablespoon dried rosemary
- ¼ teaspoon lavender
- honey (optional)

Instructions

1. Mix all ingredients in a bowl.
2. To brew hot tea: Place 1 teaspoon tea per 1 cup boiling water.
3. Let steep 5 minutes and strain.
4. Sweeten with honey.

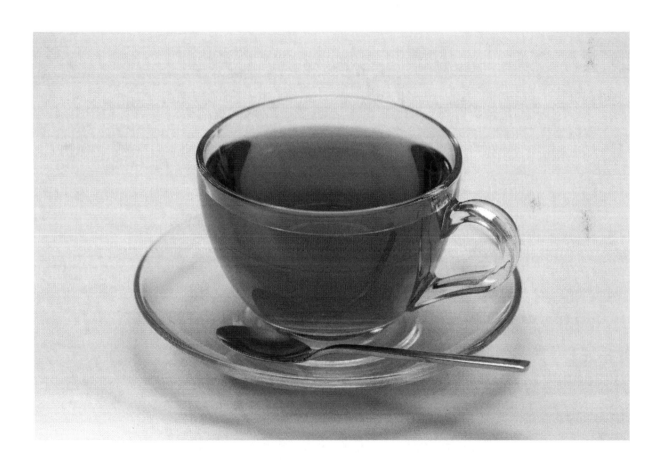

73 Purple Tea

Ingredients

- ½ cup sage leaves
- ½ cup spearmint
- 1 cup rose petals

Instructions

1. Mix all ingredients in a bowl.
2. To brew hot tea: Place 1 tablespoon tea per 1 cup boiling water.
3. Let steep 15 minutes and strain.

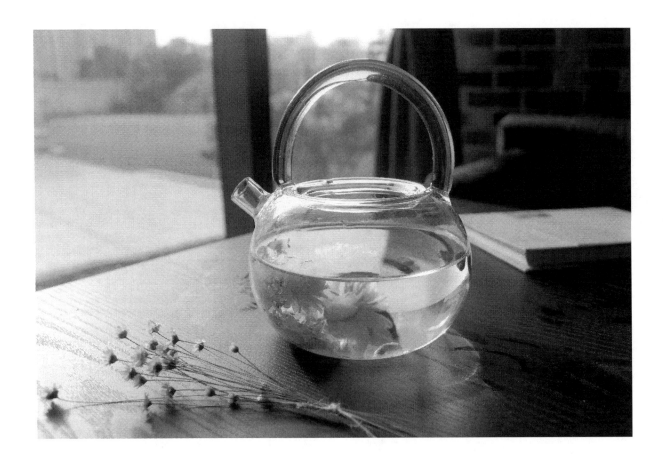

74 Heaven Tea

Ingredients

- ½ cup chamomile
- ½ cup lemon verbena
- honey (optional)
- lemon to taste

Instructions

1. Mix all ingredients in a bowl.
2. To brew hot tea: Place 1 teaspoon tea per 1 cup boiling water.
3. Let steep 7 minutes and strain.
4. Sweeten with honey.

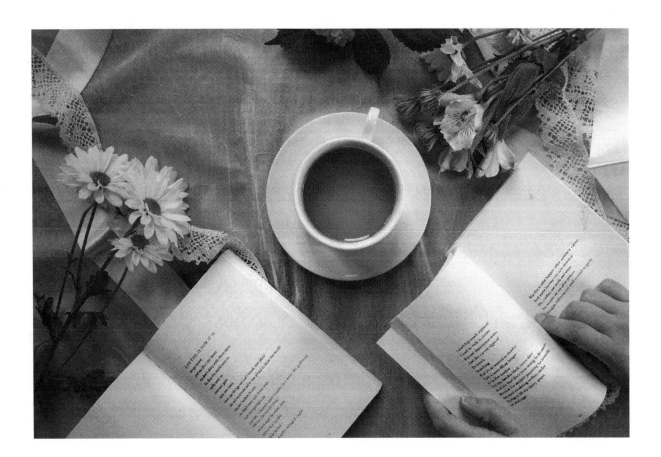

75 Sleepy Tea

Ingredients

- 1 part lavender
- 4 parts peppermint
- 1 part red raspberry leaf
- honey (optional)
- lemon to taste

Instructions

1. Mix all ingredients in a bowl.
2. To brew hot tea: Place 1 teaspoon tea per 1 cup boiling water.
3. Let steep 7 minutes and strain.
4. Sweeten with honey.

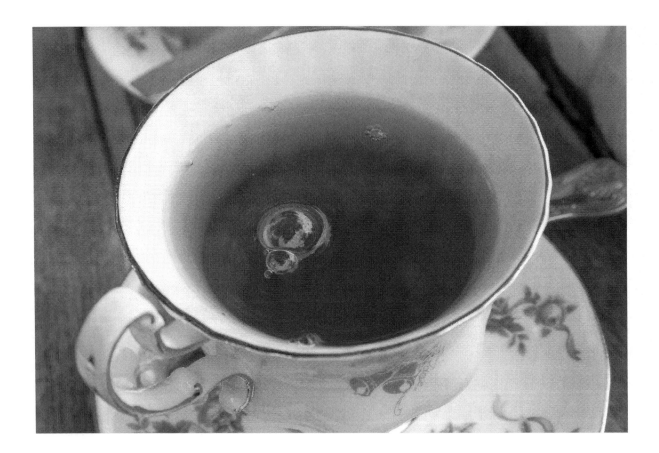

76 Chamomile Tea

Ingredients

- 1 cup chamomile
- ½ cup calendula
- ¼ part lemon peel
- 1 cup peppermint
- honey (optional)

Instructions

1. Mix all ingredients in a bowl.
2. To brew hot tea: Place 1 teaspoon tea per 1 cup boiling water.
3. Let steep 7 minutes and strain.
4. Sweeten with honey.

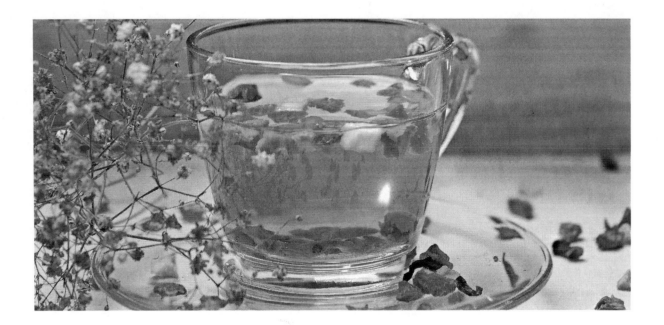

77 Sun Tea

Ingredients

- 1 tablespoon green tea leaves
- 3 whole cloves
- ¼ teaspoon ground ginger
- ½ teaspoon cinnamon
- honey (optional)

Instructions

1. Mix all ingredients in a bowl.
2. To brew hot tea: Place 1 teaspoon tea per 1 cup boiling water.
3. Let steep 5 minutes and strain.
4. Sweeten with honey.

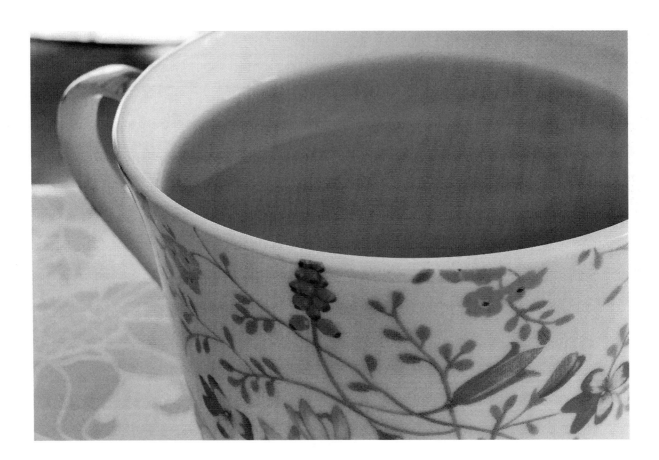

78 Moon Tea

Ingredients

- 1-inch piece dry ginger
- 3 whole cloves
- 1-ince piece cinnamon
- ½ teaspoon fennel seeds
- honey to taste

Instructions

1. Mix all ingredients in a bowl.
2. To brew hot tea: Place 1 teaspoon tea per 1 cup boiling water.
3. Let steep 5 minutes and strain.
4. Sweeten with honey.

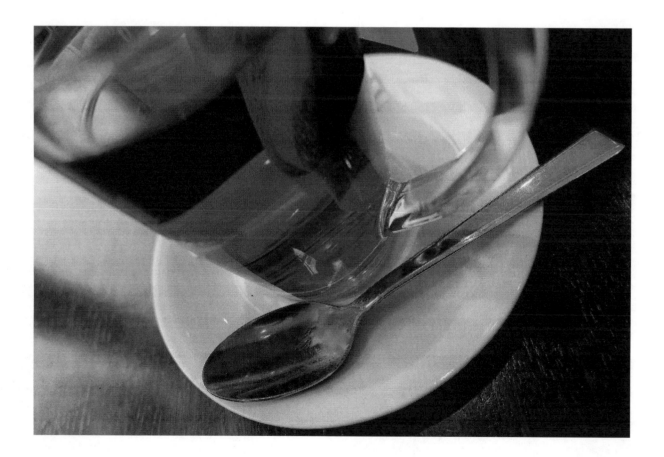

79 Herbal Tea

Ingredients

- ½ whole cinnamon stick
- 1 whole clove
- ¼ green cardamom pod
- ½ teaspoon fresh orange zest
- ½ teaspoon cut licorice root
- honey to taste

Instructions

1. Mix all ingredients in a bowl.
2. To brew hot tea: Place 1 teaspoon tea per 1 cup boiling water.
3. Let steep 8 minutes and strain.
4. Sweeten with honey.

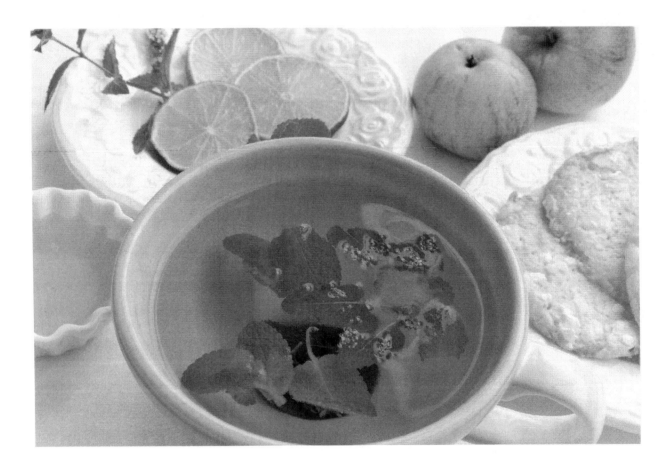

80 World Tea

Ingredients

- 1 teaspoon honey
- lemon to taste

Instructions

1. To brew hot tea: Place 1 teaspoon of honey per 1 cup boiling water.
2. Add lemon to taste.
3. Let steep 3 minutes.

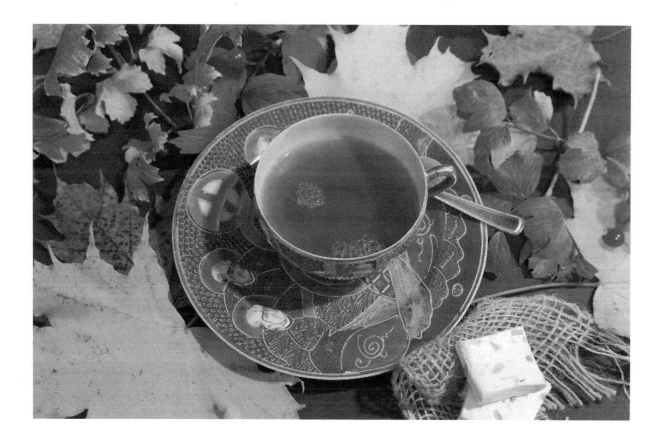

CONTENT

Made in the USA
Las Vegas, NV
08 October 2023

78745505R00037